Aphasia Workbook Daily Living

By Florence Jones

This collection of books was created for my father who has Aphasia. Over the months while working with my father on his speech therapy homework, I realized how difficult it was for him to identify the hand-drawn black and white pictures that were presented to him on his worksheets.

In the beginning I remembered the doctor telling me to make every visit a productive visit. Having a tangible book that he can take with him and one that anyone can pick up and use added consistency to his recovery.

I tried workbooks made for children, however, these seemed to insult his intelligence. I also tried computer-based speech therapy applications which were only available when he had access to a computer. He seemed to progress faster when he worked one on one with another human being.

Each page includes photographs of different items common to every day living. Also on each page are three levels of difficulty. How you choose to use each page is up to you and your patient or loved one. As I worked with my father to help him regain his speech, reading and writing, I realized the process was the same as for a child. First you learn to speak, then read, followed by writing. There are also different levels of Aphasia: one person may regain speaking very quickly while another not so quickly.

Get Started - There are three steps on each page:

Step 1 - Identify the picture: point to the picture and speak it out load. Have your patient or loved one repeat the word over and over, day after day. If your patient or loved one has severe Aphasia you might want to just do this step until your patient or loved one is able to identify the pictures. While working on this section you can reinforce the lesson by using the actual object in the picture.

Step 2 – Use the word in a sentence: this section is designed to help the patient identify the object in use. Each sentence has been chosen to help the patient regain basic sentences for every day use. Read the sentence and fill in the word. Have the patient or loved one try to verbally fill in the word own his own. He or she might need to be cued. While working on this section you can reinforce the lesson by using the actual objects.

Step 3 – Writing: after your patient or loved one has learned the objects the final step is writing the word. Have your patient write over the grayed out word, then encourage him or her to continue on their own.

Copyright 2010 by Bright Eyes Books

Hairbrush

1. Point to the picture and say the word. Then have your patient repeat the word.

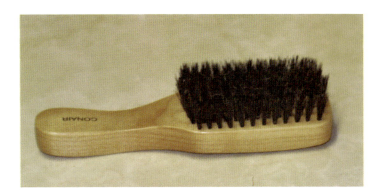

I brush my hair with a _____.

2. Read the sentence to your patient and verbally fill in the word. Read the sentence again and have your patient verbally fill in the missing word.

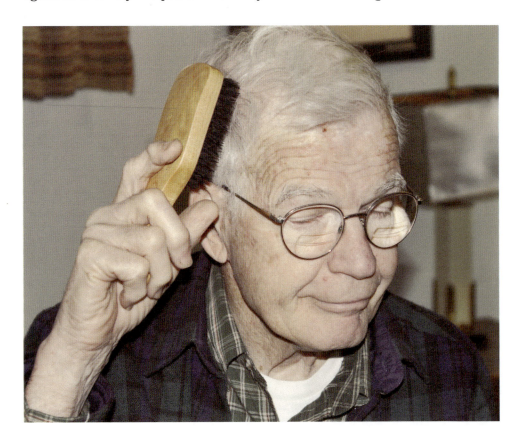

3. Have your patient practice writing the word. Trace over each shaded word then repeat the word several times on each line.

Hairbrush

Hairbrush _____

Hairbrush _____

Hairbrush _____

Hairbrush _____

Hairbrush _____

Hairbrush _____

Hairbrush _____

Hairbrush _____

Hairbrush _____

Hairbrush _____

Hairbrush _____

Hairbrush _____

Hairbrush _____

Hairbrush _____

Hairbrush _____

Hairbrush _____

Razor

1. Point to the picture and say the word. Then have your patient repeat the word.

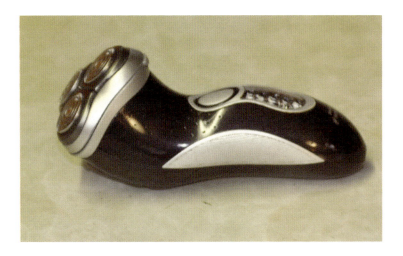

I shave with a _____.

2. Read the sentence to your patient and verbally fill in the word. Read the sentence again and have your patient verbally fill in the missing word.

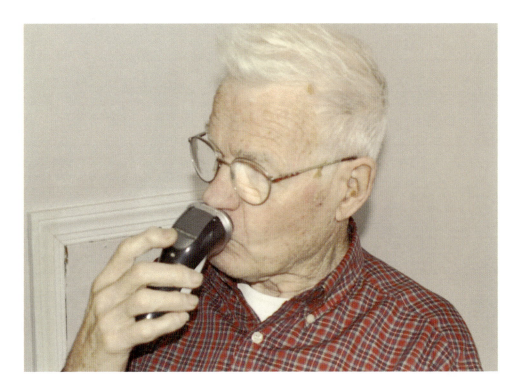

3. Have your patient practice writing the word. Trace over each shaded word then repeat the word several times on each line..

Razor

Razor _____

Razor _____

Razor _____

Razor _____

Razor _____

Razor _____

Razor _____

Razor _____

Razor _____

Razor _____

Razor _____

Razor _____

Razor _____

Razor _____

Razor _____

Medication

1. Point to the picture and say the word. Then have your patient repeat the word.

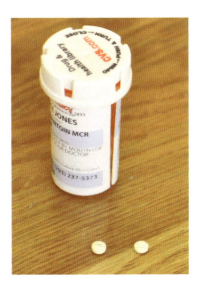

Every day I take my _____.

2. Read the sentence to your patient and verbally fill in the word. Read the sentence again and have your patient verbally fill in the missing word.

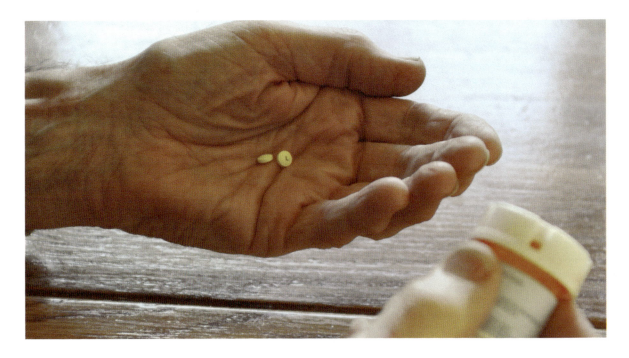

3. Have your patient practice writing the word. Trace over each shaded word then repeat the word several times on each line.

Medication

Medication _____

Medication _____

Medication _____

Medication _____

Medication _____

Medication _____

Medication _____

Medication _____

Medication _____

Medication _____

Medication _____

Medication _____

Medication _____

Medication _____

Medication _____

Toothbrush

1. Point to the picture and say the word. Then have your patient repeat the word.

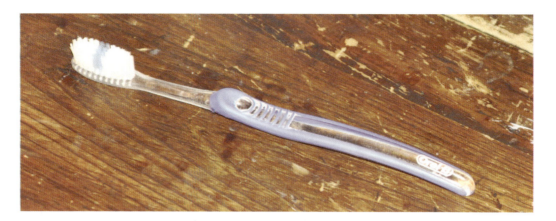

I brush my teeth with a _____.

2. Read the sentence to your patient and verbally fill in the word. Read the sentence again and have your patient verbally fill in the missing word.

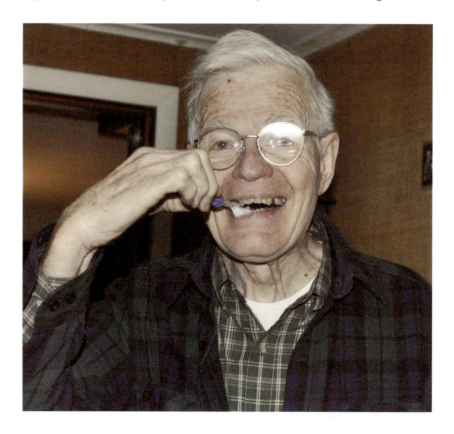

3. Have your patient practice writing the word. Trace over each shaded word then repeat the word several times on each line.

Toothbrush

Toothbrush _____

Toothbrush _____

Toothbrush _____

Toothbrush _____

Toothbrush _____

Toothbrush _____

Toothbrush _____

Toothbrush _____

Toothbrush _____

Toothbrush _____

Toothbrush _____

Toothbrush _____

Toothbrush _____

Toothbrush _____

Toothbrush _____

Toothbrush _____

Comb

1. Point to the picture and say the word. Then have your patient repeat the word.

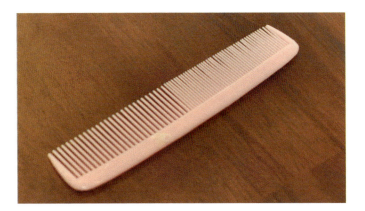

I straighten my hair with a _____.

2. Read the sentence to your patient and verbally fill in the word. Read the sentence again and have your patient verbally fill in the missing word.

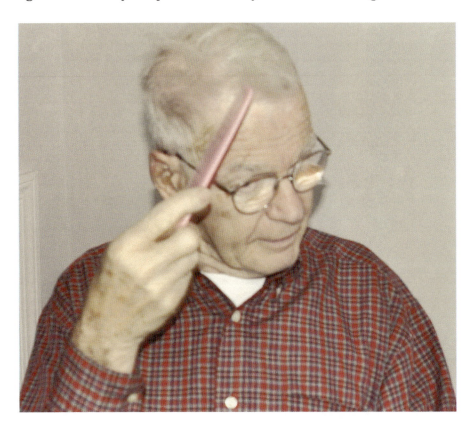

3. Have your patient practice writing the word. Trace over each shaded word then repeat the word several times on each line.

Comb

Comb _____

Comb _____

Comb _____

Comb _____

Comb _____

Comb _____

Comb _____

Comb _____

Comb _____

Comb _____

Comb _____

Comb _____

Comb _____

Comb _____

Comb _____

Soap

1. Point to the picture and say the word. Then have your patient repeat the word.

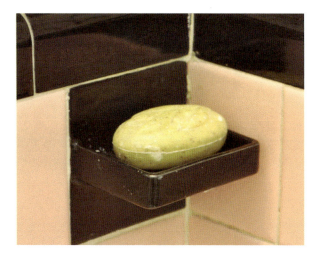

I wash my hands with _____.

2. Read the sentence to your patient and verbally fill in the word. Read the sentence again and have your patient verbally fill in the missing word.

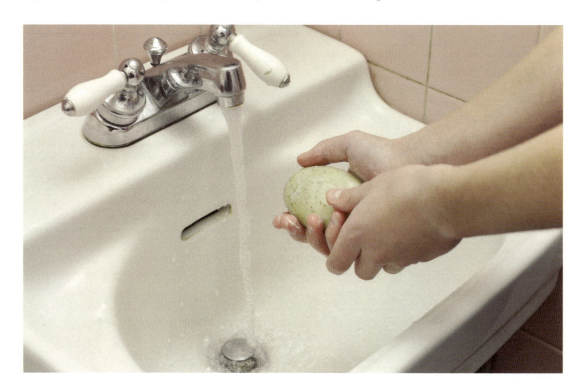

3. Have your patient practice writing the word. Trace over each shaded word then repeat the word several times on each line.

Soap

Soap _____

Soap _____

Soap _____

Soap _____

Soap _____

Soap _____

Soap _____

Soap _____

Soap _____

Soap _____

Soap _____

Soap _____

Soap _____

Soap _____

Soap _____

Bathroom

1. Point to the picture and say the word. Then have your patient repeat the word.

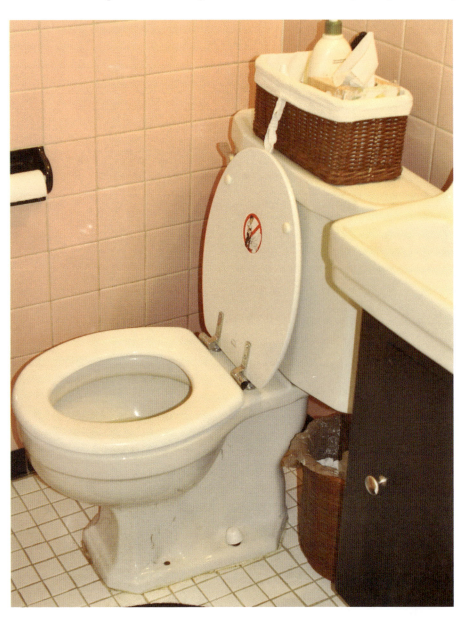

I need to use the _____.

2. Read the sentence to your patient and verbally fill in the word. Read the sentence again and have your patient verbally fill in the missing word.

3. Have your patient practice writing the word. Trace over each shaded word then repeat the word several times on each line.

Bathroom

Bathroom _____

Bathroom _____

Bathroom _____

Bathroom _____

Bathroom _____

Bathroom _____

Bathroom _____

Bathroom _____

Bathroom _____

Bathroom _____

Bathroom _____

Bathroom _____

Bathroom _____

Bathroom _____

Bathroom _____

Sink

1. Point to the picture and say the word. Then have your patient repeat the word.

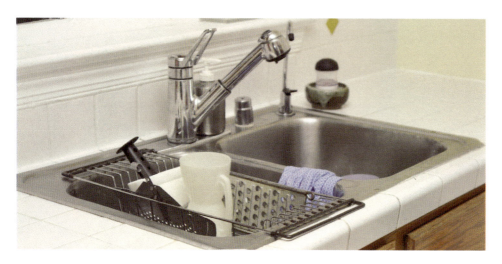

I wash my dishes in a _____.

2. Read the sentence to your patient and verbally fill in the word. Read the sentence again and have your patient verbally fill in the missing word.

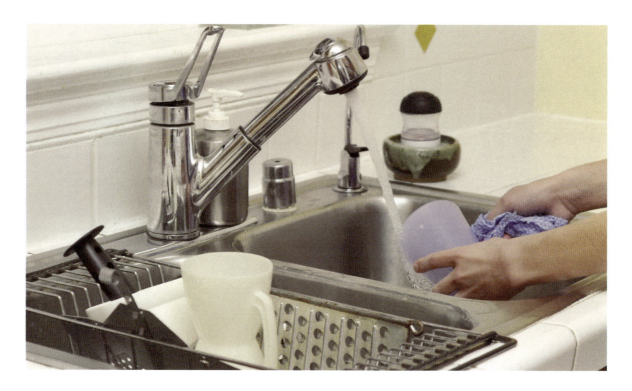

3. Have your patient practice writing the word. Trace over each shaded word then repeat the word several times on each line.

Sink

Sink _____

Sink _____

Sink _____

Sink _____

Sink _____

Sink _____

Sink _____

Sink _____

Sink _____

Sink _____

Sink _____

Sink _____

Sink _____

Sink _____

Sink _____

Sink _____

Fork

1. Point to the picture and say the word. Then have your patient repeat the word.

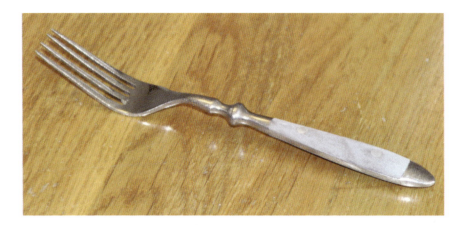

I eat with with a _____.

2. Read the sentence to your patient and verbally fill in the word. Read the sentence again and have your patient verbally fill in the missing word.

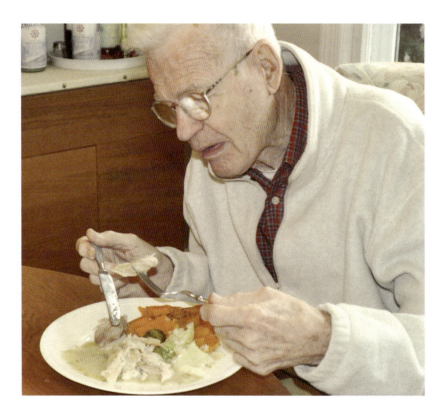

3. Have your patient practice writing the word. Trace over each shaded word then repeat the word several times on each line.

Fork

Fork _____

Fork _____

Fork _____

Fork _____

Fork _____

Fork _____

Fork _____

Fork _____

Fork _____

Fork _____

Fork _____

Fork _____

Fork _____

Fork _____

Fork _____

Fork _____

Knife

1. Point to the picture and say the word. Then have your patient repeat the word.

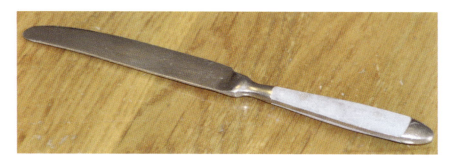

I cut my meat with a _____.

2. Read the sentence to your patient and verbally fill in the word. Read the sentence again and have your patient verbally fill in the missing word.

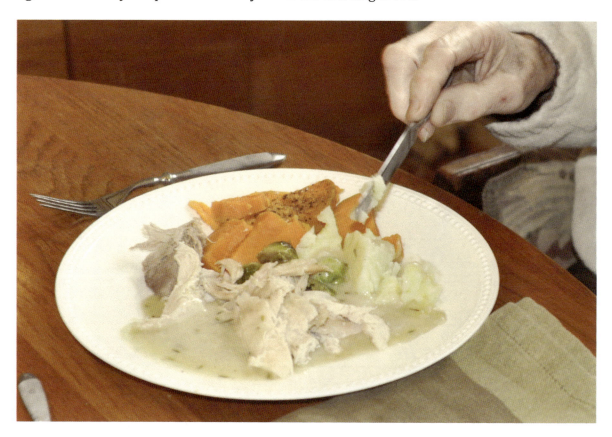

3. Have your patient practice writing the word. Trace over each shaded word then repeat the word several times on each line.

Knife

Knife _____

Knife _____

Knife _____

Knife _____

Knife _____

Knife _____

Knife _____

Knife _____

Knife _____

Knife _____

Knife _____

Knife _____

Knife _____

Knife _____

Knife _____

Cup

1. Point to the picture and say the word. Then have your patient repeat the word.

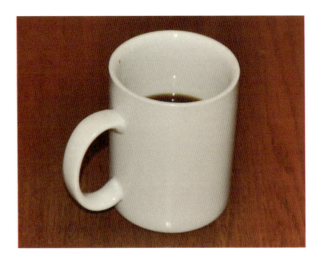

I drink my coffee from a _____.

2. Read the sentence to your patient and verbally fill in the word. Read the sentence again and have your patient verbally fill in the missing word.

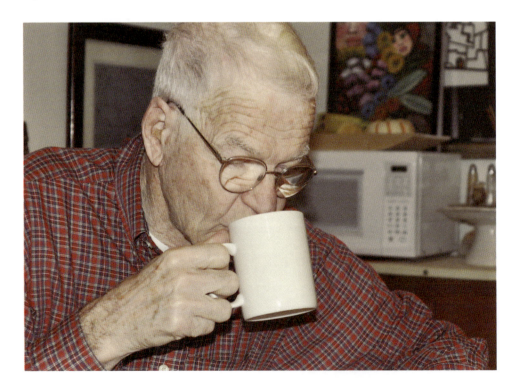

3. Have your patient practice writing the word. Trace over each shaded word then repeat the word several times on each line.

Cup

Cup _____

Cup _____

Cup _____

Cup _____

Cup _____

Cup _____

Cup _____

Cup _____

Cup _____

Cup _____

Cup _____

Cup _____

Cup _____

Cup _____

Cup _____

Glass

1. Point to the picture and say the word. Then have your patient repeat the word.

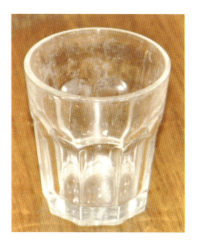

I drink my juice from a _____.

2. Read the sentence to your patient and verbally fill in the word. Read the sentence again and have your patient verbally fill in the missing word.

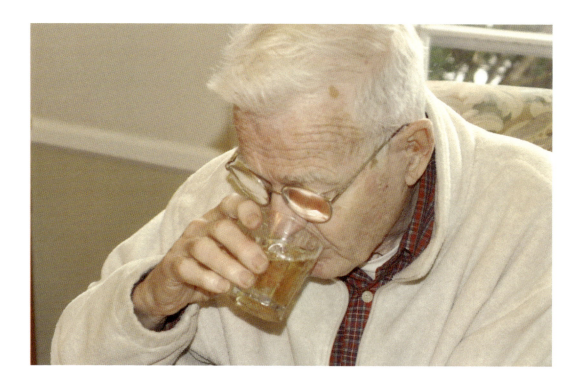

3. Have your patient practice writing the word. Trace over each shaded word then repeat the word several times on each line.

Glass

Glass _____

Glass _____

Glass _____

Glass _____

Glass _____

Glass _____

Glass _____

Glass _____

Glass _____

Glass _____

Glass _____

Glass _____

Glass _____

Glass _____

Glass _____

Microwave

1. Point to the picture and say the word. Then have your patient repeat the word.

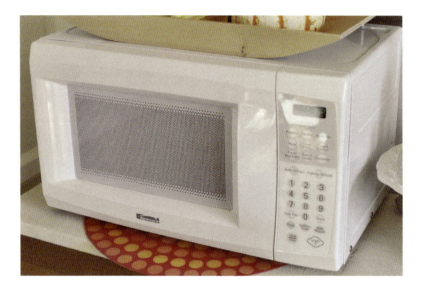

I heat my coffee in a _____.

2. Read the sentence to your patient and verbally fill in the word. Read the sentence again and have your patient verbally fill in the missing word.

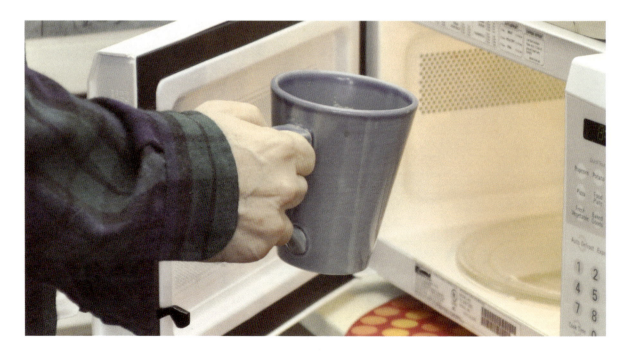

3. Have your patient practice writing the word. Trace over each shaded word then repeat the word several times on each line.

Microwave

Microwave _____

Microwave _____

Microwave _____

Microwave _____

Microwave _____

Microwave _____

Microwave _____

Microwave _____

Microwave _____

Microwave _____

Microwave _____

Microwave _____

Microwave _____

Microwave _____

Microwave _____

Microwave _____

Frying Pan

1. Point to the picture and say the word. Then have your patient repeat the word.

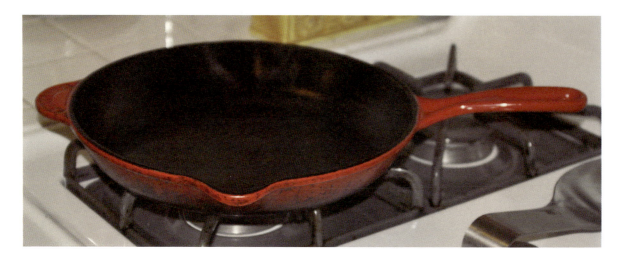

I cook my eggs in a _____.

2. Read the sentence to your patient and verbally fill in the word. Read the sentence again and have your patient verbally fill in the missing word.

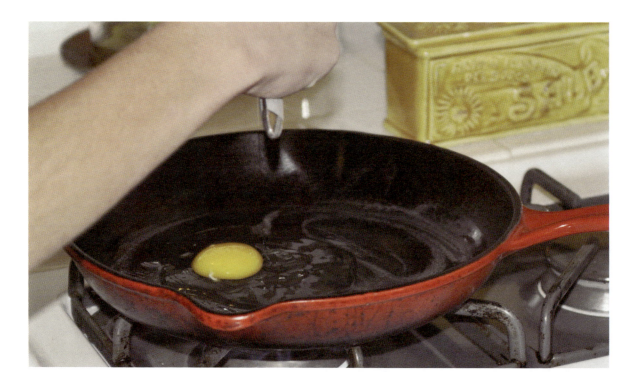

3. Have your patient practice writing the word. Trace over each shaded word then repeat the word several times on each line.

Frying Pan

Frying Pan_____

Frying Pan_____

Frying Pan_____

Frying Pan_____

Frying Pan_____

Frying Pan_____

Frying Pan_____

Frying Pan_____

Frying Pan_____

Frying Pan_____

Frying Pan_____

Frying Pan_____

Frying Pan_____

Frying Pan_____

Frying Pan_____

Lid

1. Point to the picture and say the word. Then have your patient repeat the word.

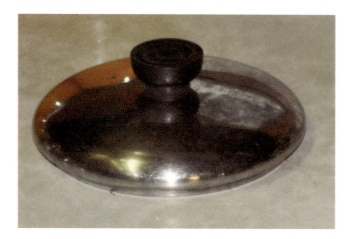

The sauce pan has a _____.

2. Read the sentence to your patient and verbally fill in the word. Read the sentence again and have your patient verbally fill in the missing word.

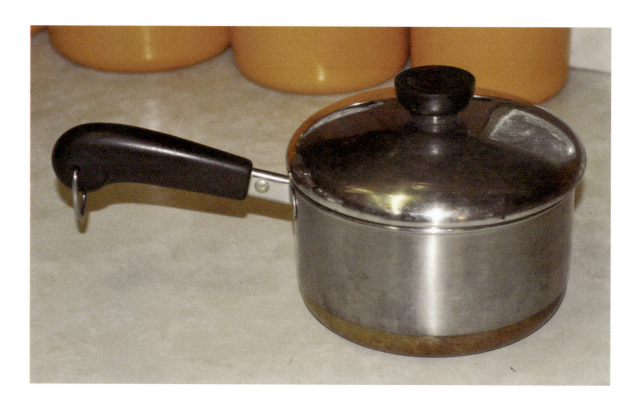

3. Have your patient practice writing the word. Trace over each shaded word then repeat the word several times on each line.

Lid

Lid _____

Lid _____

Lid _____

Lid _____

Lid _____

Lid _____

Lid _____

Lid _____

Lid _____

Lid _____

Lid _____

Lid _____

Lid _____

Lid _____

Lid _____

Table

1. Point to the picture and say the word. Then have your patient repeat the word.

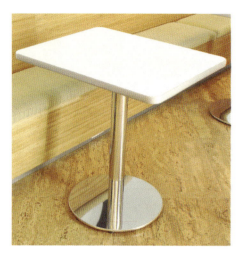

I sit at a _____.

2. Read the sentence to your patient and verbally fill in the word. Read the sentence again and have your patient verbally fill in the missing word.

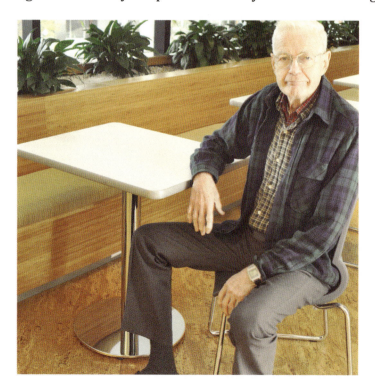

3. Have your patient practice writing the word. Trace over each shaded word then repeat the word several times on each line.

Table

Table _____

Table _____

Table _____

Table _____

Table _____

Table _____

Table _____

Table _____

Table _____

Table _____

Table _____

Table _____

Table _____

Table _____

Table _____

Plate

1. Point to the picture and say the word. Then have your patient repeat the word.

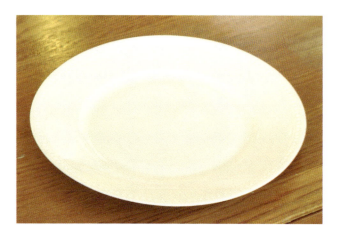

I eat food from a _____.

2. Read the sentence to your patient and verbally fill in the word. Read the sentence again and have your patient verbally fill in the missing word.

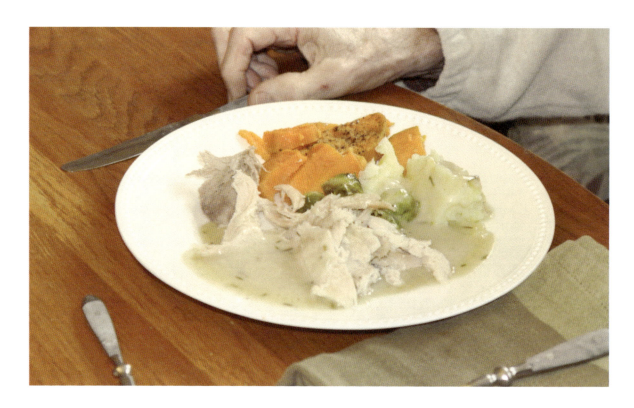

3. Have your patient practice writing the word. Trace over each shaded word then repeat the word several times on each line.

Plate

Plate _____

Plate _____

Plate _____

Plate _____

Plate _____

Plate _____

Plate _____

Plate _____

Plate _____

Plate _____

Plate _____

Plate _____

Plate _____

Plate _____

Plate _____

Sauce Pan

1. Point to the picture and say the word. Then have your patient repeat the word.

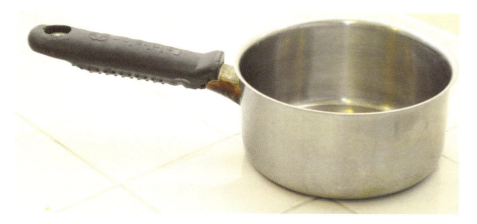

I cook my oatmeal in a _____.

2. Read the sentence to your patient and verbally fill in the word. Read the sentence again and have your patient verbally fill in the missing word.

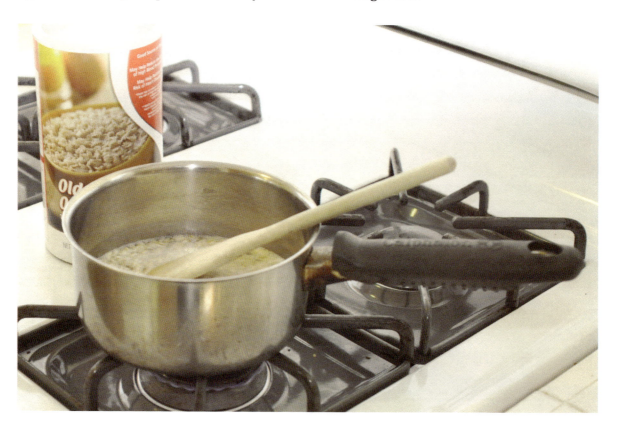

3. Have your patient practice writing the word. Trace over each shaded word then repeat the word several times on each line.

Sauce Pan

Sauce Pan _____

Sauce Pan _____

Sauce Pan _____

Sauce Pan _____

Sauce Pan _____

Sauce Pan _____

Sauce Pan _____

Sauce Pan _____

Sauce Pan _____

Sauce Pan _____

Sauce Pan _____

Sauce Pan _____

Sauce Pan _____

Sauce Pan _____

Sauce Pan _____

Bowl

1. Point to the picture and say the word. Then have your patient repeat the word.

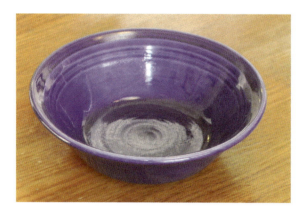

I eat my cereal from a _____.

2. Read the sentence to your patient and verbally fill in the word. Read the sentence again and have your patient verbally fill in the missing word.

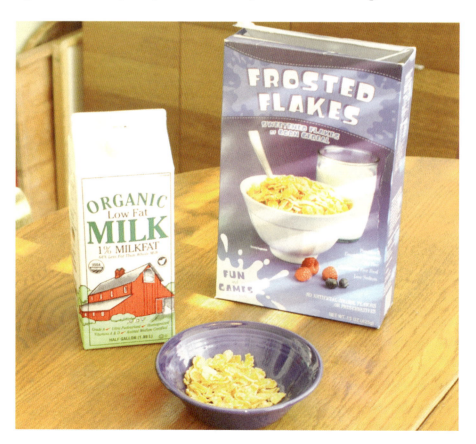

3. Have your patient practice writing the word. Trace over each shaded word then repeat the word several times on each line.

Bowl

Bowl _____

Bowl _____

Bowl _____

Bowl _____

Bowl _____

Bowl _____

Bowl _____

Bowl _____

Bowl _____

Bowl _____

Bowl _____

Bowl _____

Bowl _____

Bowl _____

Bowl _____

Spoon

1. Point to the picture and say the word. Then have your patient repeat the word.

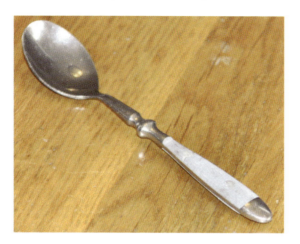

I eat my oatmeal with a _____.

2. Read the sentence to your patient and verbally fill in the word. Read the sentence again and have your patient verbally fill in the missing word.

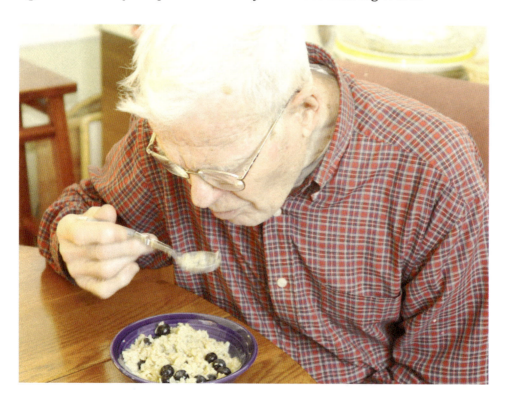

3. Have your patient practice writing the word. Trace over each shaded word then repeat the word several times on each line.

Spoon

Spoon _____

Spoon _____

Spoon _____

Spoon _____

Spoon _____

Spoon _____

Spoon _____

Spoon _____

Spoon _____

Spoon _____

Spoon _____

Spoon _____

Spoon _____

Spoon _____

Spoon _____

Napkin

1. Point to the picture and say the word. Then have your patient repeat the word.

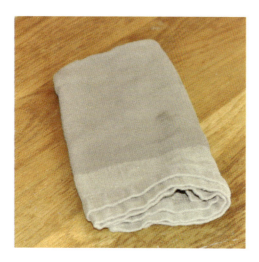

I wipe my mouth with a _____.

2. Read the sentence to your patient and verbally fill in the word. Read the sentence again and have your patient verbally fill in the missing word.

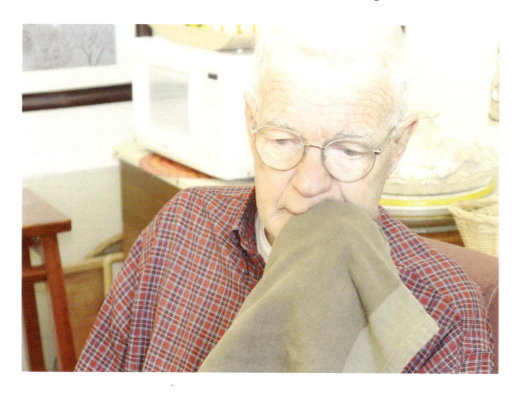

3. Have your patient practice writing the word. Trace over each shaded word then repeat the word several times on each line.

Napkin

Napkin _____

Napkin _____

Napkin _____

Napkin _____

Napkin _____

Napkin _____

Napkin _____

Napkin _____

Napkin _____

Napkin _____

Napkin _____

Napkin _____

Napkin _____

Napkin _____

Napkin _____

Toaster

1. Point to the picture and say the word. Then have your patient repeat the word.

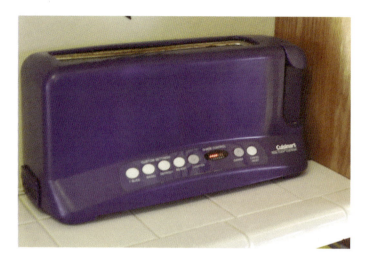

I toast my bread in a _____.

2. Read the sentence to your patient and verbally fill in the word. Read the sentence again and have your patient verbally fill in the missing word.

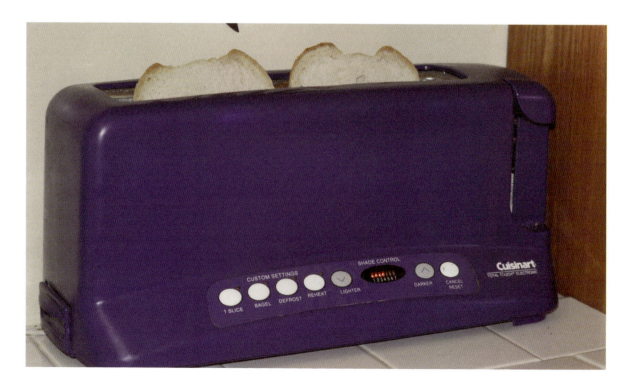

3. Have your patient practice writing the word. Trace over each shaded word then repeat the word several times on each line.

Toaster

Toaster _____

Toaster _____

Toaster _____

Toaster _____

Toaster _____

Toaster _____

Toaster _____

Toaster _____

Toaster _____

Toaster _____

Toaster _____

Toaster _____

Toaster _____

Toaster _____

Toaster _____

Book

1. Point to the picture and say the word. Then have your patient repeat the word.

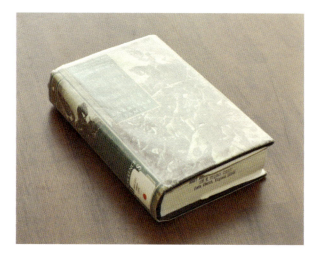

I read a _____.

2. Read the sentence to your patient and verbally fill in the word. Read the sentence again and have your patient verbally fill in the missing word.

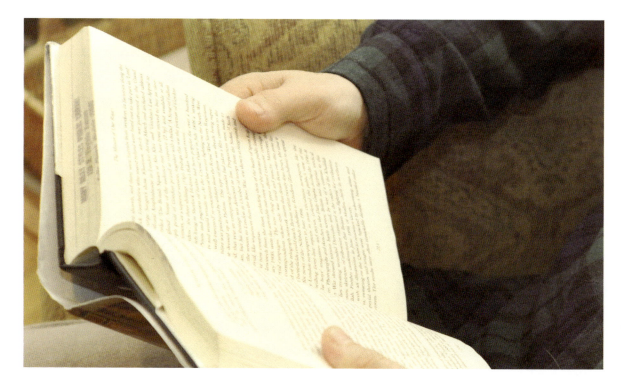

3. Have your patient practice writing the word. Trace over each shaded word then repeat the word several times on each line.

Book

Book_____

Book_____

Book_____

Book_____

Book_____

Book_____

Book_____

Book_____

Book_____

Book_____

Book_____

Book_____

Book_____

Book_____

Book_____

Watch

1. Point to the picture and say the word. Then have your patient repeat the word.

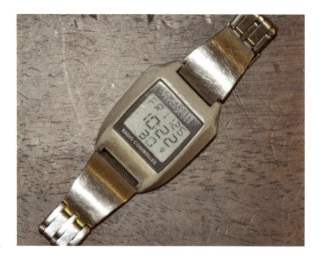

I check the time on my _____.

2. Read the sentence to your patient and verbally fill in the word. Read the sentence again and have your patient verbally fill in the missing word.

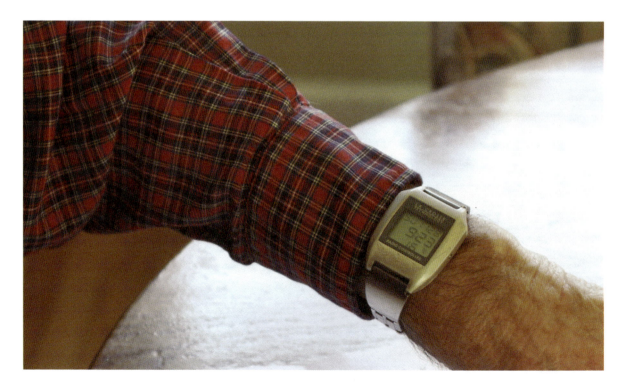

3. Have your patient practice writing the word. Trace over each shaded word then repeat the word several times on each line.

Watch

Watch _____

Watch _____

Watch _____

Watch _____

Watch _____

Watch _____

Watch _____

Watch _____

Watch _____

Watch _____

Watch _____

Watch _____

Watch _____

Watch _____

Watch _____

Alphabet

Aa	Ii	Qq	Yy
Bb	Jj	Rr	Zz
Cc	Kk	Ss	
Dd	Ll	Tt	
Ee	Mm	Uu	
Ff	Nn	Vv	
Gg	Oo	Ww	
Hh	Pp	Xx	

Numbers

1	11	10	100
2	12	20	200
3	13	30	300
4	14	40	400
5	15	50	500
6	16	60	600
7	17	70	700
8	18	80	800
9	19	90	900
10	20	100	1000

Dedicated to my father
David Jones

This series of Aphasia Workbooks is available for purchase at
www.amazon.com or www.createspace.com (for larger quantities)

Made in the USA
Lexington, KY
20 November 2014